Making the Most of My Second Chance

Making the Most of My Second Chance

RONALD SCHOEN

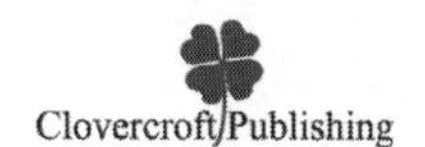

Making the Most of My Second Chance

Published by Carpenter's Son Publishing, Franklin, Tennessee

Published in association with Larry Carpenter of
Christian Book Services, LLC
www.christianbookservices.com

Edited by David Brown

Interior layout by Suzanne Lawing

Cover design by Julie Baltes

Printed in the United States of America

978-1-952025-73-0

DEDICATION

In memory of my nephew Caleb Kunkle and Scott Dippold.

In memory, also, of those who have suffered from or died from cancer.

CONTENTS

"I can do all things through him who strengthens me."
(Phil. 4:13)

PROLOGUE

"Tina, you've gotta get me out of here. I'm gonna die."

A few minutes later, I was in a medevac van on my way to another hospital. It was a rough ride. I joked with my father later that the vehicle must have had square tires, but I wasn't in any state to make light of the matter at the time. I was bleeding profusely and in severe pain despite a potent cocktail of painkilling meds coursing through my veins.

I thought it was the end for me.

***

A week before, a minor surgery to remove a polyp in my colon had gone terribly wrong. I was only forty-three years old, but I knew my unhealthy lifestyle put me at risk. Hoping to avoid the cancer that had plagued my family, I went in for a colonoscopy. A follow-up, routine surgery was set up to take out the golf ball-sized growth that, my doctor asserted, was not cancerous.

When I woke up, however, I didn't feel well. It was normal, the nurses said reassuringly. A week later, I was speeding toward a more advanced medical center, hoping to stay alive long enough to undergo an emergency surgery to repair the damage caused by the first one. The knife used to cut out the polyp had nicked my bowel, and I was being poisoned by the contents of my own body.

When I arrived at the new hospital, there wasn't much life in me, but I was still on this side of the great divide. Then something happened. It was the strangest, most wonderful thing I've ever experienced. It's hard to explain, and I'm still trying to figure it all out. But one thing I know: the experience of that day changed my life.

Some names in this book have been modified

Chapter 1

THE BACKGROUND

My parents were my role models. They weren't perfect, but they instilled in me the core pieces of my identity: Catholic faith, hard work, and committed marriage. Throughout my life, I've tried to live up to these ideals.

Growing Up in God's Country

I'm the second youngest of six children: two girls and four boys. My mom was the oldest of twelve and my dad was the second youngest of four—but only by a couple of minutes. Yes, Dad has an identical twin.

Mom grew up on a farm in Fort Recovery, a small town on the western edge of Ohio near the Indiana line. The town takes its name from the military installation built there in the late eighteenth century. General "Mad" Anthony Wayne fought there before the Treaty of Greenville brought peace between white Americans and Indians and opened up the area to white settlement.

German Catholics poured into Mercer County in the mid-eighteenth century, buying up the fertile farmland. Their legacy is still obvious in the many impressive structures that give the area its nickname, "Land of the Cross-Tipped Churches."

Mom's family lived off their land. They raised a few cows, which provided milk. They also raised a few chickens. I remember, when I was young, watching my grandpa, grandma, aunts, uncles, mom, and dad butcher them. I was the "gizzard guy," tasked with extracting that organ from the freshly slaughtered birds. It wasn't my favorite job in the world, but it was just part of life in my family. Grandma and Grandpa also had a huge garden and apple and pear trees. They got very few things from the stores in town.

My mother's family were and still are an extremely close, loving family. Grandpa passed away roughly twenty years ago from a heart attack, and Grandma passed away fifteen years later. She lived through two strokes and breast, colon, and kidney cancer in the ninety-six years she was with us. Unfortunately, my grandma also had to live through every parent's worst nightmare, the death of a child. My mom's younger sister, Doris, passed away from pancreatic cancer a few years prior to Grandma's death.

On my dad's side, my grandpa was also a farmer. Grandma Schoen was a homemaker. They too lived in Fort Recovery, just down the road from where Mom and Dad live, which is only a few miles away from where my maternal grandparents lived. Grandpa Schoen died at age eighty-four of an aneurysm. Grandma, who had survived breast cancer and lived with Parkinson's, died a few years after Grandpa.

I remember riding my bike over to their house almost weekly to hang out with them when I was young. I'll never forget Grandma baking sugar cookies with multicolored icing. They were amazing!

Unfortunately, I don't remember much about Dad's oldest sibling, Bernice, as an aneurysm took her life when I was very young. Dad also lost his oldest brother at an early age. Lester passed away at age twenty-four from colon cancer, shortly after he got out of the Army and had joined the National Guard.

In addition to their Catholic faith, the Germans who settled Mercer County also brought a strong work ethic. Anyone raised in the area is bound to absorb it, and I was no exception. This ethic was passed on to me as I grew up in our country home outside Fort Recovery in the 1970s. I was about ten years old when Dad got me a job picking up beer and pop cans at a bar down the road from our house. Sometimes, one of my brothers helped. Six mornings a week, from 6:00 to 6:30, I walked around the outside of the bar and its parking lot, picking up the discarded cans. On Saturday mornings, there were heaps of them—fifteen to twenty bags' worth. I'd pile them up at home, and on Saturday mornings, I'd crush them; sometimes with my feet, sometimes with a sledgehammer. Dad gave me all of the money earned by recycling the cans, except for a few dollars he kept for gas. Like a good entrepreneur, I invested some of my earnings in a capital improvement to improve efficiency. When I had enough money, I bought a can smasher. That was a great day!

Mom would let me keep a few dollars for spending money, but she made sure that all the rest went into a savings account. This was the German way: hard work and thrift. I would use those savings when I was a teenager to buy my first car, a 1983 T-Bird. It was a beautiful car. But it was also a lemon, requiring continuous repairs. My dad got tired of dealing with it. One day, I came home, and it was gone. He had sold it.

My brother and I also mowed grass and shoveled snow for our parish church, St. Paul's, one of the historic "cross-tipped churches," located southeast of Fort Recovery in the unincorporated community of Sharpsburg. The church was just up the road from our home. Practicing our faith was a part of life, as it was for most in our tight-knit community. My three brothers and I all assisted at the altar as Mass servers, and my dad helped out as an usher. My mom prepared meals at funerals and counted offertory money. I enjoyed being around the church and chatting with our priests. There were a few occasions when we got a last-minute call from our friends (and neighbors) to substitute as servers for their boys. Their cows were out, and they needed to chase them down!

Confronting Death

As you can see, mine was a quintessentially small-town-America upbringing, with lots of friends and family around. Family, church, school, and work pretty much defined existence. It was a good life, but it also had its hardships.

When I was in my early teens, my neighbor Rick, who was in his early twenties, was involved in a terrible car accident. Even after he was released from the hospital, his road to recovery was long and difficult. Members of my family would walk through the neighbors' field to Rick's mom's house. There, my parents and older siblings helped Rick's mother "pattern" him, while my younger brother and I washed the van of Rick's caregiver. Patterning is a method for getting your fingers, toes, and other body parts to send signals to your brain in order to try to get everything working together again. Rick's caregiver, Joan, was a wonderful woman—a blessing from God.

When I got older and stronger, I began to help pattern Rick as well. Joan always corrected me when I wasn't doing something exactly the way she wanted it done, which I understood and respected. Helping Rick was one of the most eye-opening and humbling things I ever had the honor to be involved in. It helped me see how we tend to take simple things for granted—a lesson I would revisit when my own health crisis occurred.

Rick passed away from cancer about the same time we lost my nephew Caleb. In 2016, when Caleb was seventeen years old and starting his senior year of high school, he was driving to football practice on his first day of school when he lost control of his vehicle and nearly died. As a result of his injuries, he became paralyzed from the sternum down. Even so, Caleb continued to be an active and beloved part of our family. So, we were all stunned when Caleb passed away on June 19, 2019.

Rick and Caleb had been friends, and both were extremely ornery. Rick's caretaker, Joan, runs a neurological center, and Caleb worked there while he and Rick were in therapy. The two of them hit it off and enjoyed goofing off together. Caleb would give other kids rides on his lap as he drove his wheelchair around the place. His and Rick's high spirits made life interesting. Anyone who got to know either of them became a better person.

Bats, Eggs, and My First Real Job

I walked to school from the first through sixth grades. The school was right beside the church, which was just a short walk around the corner from our home. My friends and I would sometimes get volunteered for "bat patrol," which meant taking up our tennis rackets and trying to rid the old elementary school building of its unwelcomed inhabitants. My mom joined the staff as the assistant cook as soon as my younger brother was old enough to go to school. He's only a week shy of two years younger than I am. Our main cook was my neighbor Rick's mom, Mary. From fourth through sixth grade, it wasn't unusual for my mom to volunteer me to help out in the kitchen during my lunchtime, cleaning uneaten food off trays. I wasn't a big fan of that job because I selfishly wanted to play with my friends at recess.

After the sixth grade, I went to the junior/senior high school in Fort Recovery, where I played basketball and baseball. Following graduation, I went to ITT Technical Institute (ITT), a technical school in Dayton that no longer exists. My original plan had been to go into accounting, as I loved working with numbers. But when my brother started working in construction, I thought it would be great if I could collaborate with him by handling the design side of things. So, I opted for architecture. Dad wasn't thrilled about my going to college, but Mom was supportive and agreed to assist with an interest-free loan. For two years, I studied architecture year-round at ITT. I lived in Dayton during the week and came home on the weekends to work. During those weekends, I worked at the same bar where I had picked up cans as a kid. But I had graduated to bigger things. Now I tended bar!

I also packed eggs on Saturday and Sunday mornings and again in the afternoons. The couple I worked for, Steve and Mary Ann, were people sent to me from God. I can't say enough about them. I was grateful to have the paying work, but that wasn't the main benefit. What I really enjoyed was when they stopped by just to see how I was doing at school and in life in general. Steve is now a retired banker while Mary Ann continues to run the chicken house. We are still very close friends to this day. Part of the reason that we remain good friends is that we see one another at church on occasion. I usually see them whenever there's a Mass for my nephew Caleb at their church. They and my oldest sister, Kathy (Caleb's mom), are members of the same parish.

While I was going to college, bartending, and packing eggs, I made time for fun by playing softball with my friends at local fields. It was just a "beer league" brand of ball, but for a while I was seriously committed to it, sometimes playing seven days a week as I anchored the middle of the defense as shortstop or second baseman. I absolutely loved hanging out with my buddies and playing softball, and continued doing so for the next nineteen years.

After graduating from the tech school that I went to for two years, I got a job at the local lumber yard where I did some design work—primarily on houses—and loaded some trucks. I worked there for roughly fifteen months. I was employed at a couple other places over the next two years, then went to a nearby architecture and engineering firm where I started working on commercial projects. I was there for six and a half years.

Falling in Love on 9/11

Through the late 1990s and early 2000s, I was single, working my architecture job, and living in a small (650 square feet), two-story, two-bedroom home in Coldwater, a town about fifteen miles east of Fort Recovery. For fun, I continued to play softball, which is where I met Charles. He worked at a local factory that produced health care equipment. One day, Charles introduced me to a woman he worked with. Tina had been married before, and she had a two-year-old son, Adam. Her first husband had been abusive toward her, so Tina fled the marriage to protect them both.

The date of our first meeting is easy to remember: September 11, 2001. Both of us had been so busy working that day that we had not yet heard the news from New York and Washington. After getting off work, Tina and Adam came over to my house. I had just finished mowing the lawn and was not looking my best, but I guess Tina was able to look past that. When we went inside, I flipped on the TV and we saw the news.

Tina was a pretty, fun-loving, family driven, and hard-working lady. I found all of these qualities attractive, and our relationship gradually took off. Throughout our time dating, we both did a lot of thinking. She had to determine whether she could trust another man after her first marriage took such a bad turn, and I had to figure out whether she would ever trust another man—

not to mention, whether I could be a good, loving stepfather to her son.

I grew up babysitting kids, so I had no objection to helping her parent Adam as if he were my own. More difficult was Tina's marital situation. I struggled over whether I could marry a woman who was divorced. It wasn't that I was judgmental toward her; it was more that I was confused and mystified by the prospect. The whole situation was completely new to me. I saw my parents argue at times, but the thought of them ever getting divorced never even entered my mind. There was never a thought that they didn't love one another. So, to say I was ignorant about the entire situation is an understatement.

Over the course of the period we dated, there were times that I questioned whether I was doing the right thing by dating a divorced woman. One day, I went to my parents' house for a visit and simply asked them if they approved of my dating a divorced mother with a son. We discussed it for a while. At the end of the discussion, they asked me if I loved them. Of course, I told them that I did. Then I asked them whether they thought God would be alright with me potentially marrying her someday and becoming an instant father. They told me they'd support whatever decision I made.

I remember them telling me that if I was uncertain of what God would think, I should go to church and ask God, so I did that. One day, I went into St. Paul's, knelt down, and asked God what he thought about a future for Tina and me. As is usually the case, there were no voices or visions, but I had peace that I was going down the right path.

Even though I wasn't devout in my faith at the time, it was important for me to stay in the good graces of the Church and to center my relationship with Tina and Adam around the Church. Tina wasn't Catholic at the time, but had gone to church when she was young, thanks to a neighbor who took her. Her mom, dad, and brothers never went to church. After many months of dating, Tina kindly agreed to become Catholic so as to root our unity more deeply in a common faith. Her willingness to take that step was one thing that convinced me that our relationship could last. We went through Rite of Christian Initiation of Adults classes together and she was received into the Church at the Easter Vigil in 2004.

On October 2, 2004, we were married at Holy Trinity Catholic Church in Coldwater. I was both thrilled and nervous. I had always wanted a family, and now I felt like that dream was coming to fruition. As was the custom in our rural community, it was a big wedding. I'll never forget the wedding Mass. Right before the ceremony, the celebrant asked my best man, Jake, if he had the ring. Neither one of us had it. Apparently, Tina had taken the rings the previous evening and hadn't told me. So, we ended up getting married with a different ring. After the Mass, Tina's matron of honor gave me my wedding ring and Father blessed it. Needless to say,

I haven't taken it off since—nor have I heard the end of it sixteen years later (and counting).

Our New Household

Our married life began in my little house in Coldwater, but we soon outgrew it. In 2006, Tina and I had a son, Troy. The house was too small for the four of us, so we started looking for a larger place. By this time, I had been working for my current company, another architectural firm, for several years. My primary responsibility had been designing cabinetry, especially for school buildings. Tina continued to work at her factory job.

We debated where we should try to find a home. Tina wanted to move back to the town where she was raised, thirty miles to the south, and I wanted to move back to my hometown, fifteen miles west. Unable to agree, we decided to stay in Coldwater. Since we were both raised in the country, we decided to find something outside town.

We struggled to find a house for sale. With my background in architecture and one of my brothers being in construction, we thought we might build a house. So, we looked for land. Once again, no luck. So, we resorted to our last option: knocking on doors and asking people if they would consider selling their homes. Still, no luck. Then, a few weeks after we'd given up on that approach, one of the houses we knocked on became available. The reason was a sad one—the couple was getting a divorce—but the result was fortunate for us. We purchased the home.

While we were grateful to have our place in the country, the episode was a stressful one. After we signed the papers to take ownership, we rented the home to the divorced mother and her five children for an additional month. At the same time, we signed a contract to sell our original house to a newly married couple. As a result, we had roughly a month to fix up the new home for us to move into before we had to be out of our old house.

So, while Tina was taking care of Adam and Troy every night after she returned from her factory job, I would go to the new house after my office job and remove carpet, install drywall, cut and stain trim, and a host of other tasks. Needless to say, we were both extremely tired through this period, and eager to move into our new home when the busy month was over.

After the move, we settled into a normal routine. Tina and I continued to work while we hired someone to babysit the boys. The care provider lived in town, close to the school. This was convenient because Adam could walk to her house after school. Most weekends, we went to church as a family.

Seventeen months to the day after Troy was born, we had our second son together, Clayton. We had been blessed with three healthy boys. While we were ecstatic over this addition to our family, the pregnancy was difficult for Tina. She developed kidney problems and other complications. Our doctor told us that we could continue expanding our family, but there would definitely be quite a bit of risk involved for Tina and any additional children. We always wanted a little girl, but we didn't want to take any serious risks with Tina's health. So, after discussing it at great length and praying about it, we made the extremely difficult decision to prevent us from having any more children.

With our good jobs, new home, and thriving family, it may have appeared on the surface that our family was doing well. In some respects, we were. But problems were bubbling just beneath the surface. Although I prayed and practiced the basics of my Catholic faith, I see now that I needed to be drawn closer to God and to become aware of His intimate involvement in my life. I know that this often happens through struggle and suffering. Both were on my horizon.

Chapter 2

THE STRUGGLE

It was about seven years ago that things started to unravel at home.

It's hard to say exactly what went wrong. Much of it had to do with the normal stresses of life and my failure to handle them in healthy ways. Adam was moving through his teenage years, taking on more activities and exploring the limits of discipline, as most teens do. As our sons grew up, there were additional expenses, and the financial burden began to weigh on me. Work had lost its freshness and interest and became more drudgery than fulfilment. In the face of these challenges, instead of pulling together, Tina and I pushed each other away. We began to argue more frequently. Instead of being supportive, we became another cross for each other to bear.

Surveys show that finances are one of the most common causes of marital tension, and I've certainly seen that firsthand. Tina's first husband had spent irresponsibly, so she entered the marriage with concerns about finances. Tina and I also had different upbringings with different attitudes toward money and possessions. These are normal issues that couples need to deal with, but we simply failed to resolve them in a fruitful way.

Things Go Bad

In response to these stresses, I made poor decisions. I had played softball for nineteen years. It was a healthy way to let off steam, get good physical exercise, and was a source of camaraderie as I formed and maintained friendships with other guys. As I got older, busier, and family life got even more hectic, I decided to quit playing softball. It was a reasonable decision in some ways, but it also cut me off from relationships and activities that had helped me cope with life.

Much more detrimental were my personal vices. I had already been a smoker for years. Now I started to drink. It began with a few beers once in a while, then became a few beers virtually every night. The worse it got in the house, the more I separated myself from the situation altogether and went outside to work—and to smoke and drink. Sometimes, our boys would come out and we'd play sports or hang out together, but mostly my outside time was simply an avoidance of problems I couldn't face in the house. It was wrong and I knew it was wrong, but that's what I did.

Funding my bad habits obviously didn't do anything to alleviate our financial challenges, nor did it help our marriage. Tina's ex-husband had been a drinker as well, and when he drank, he cheated on her. This quite understandably added to her negative reaction to my drinking. She would accuse me of being unfaithful, which aggravated my hostility toward her. I was never unfaithful to her, and with God's help, I never will be. I take my wedding vows too seriously to contemplate that. But given her experience, I can't blame her for being upset and suspicious.

A vicious cycle developed. Tina began calling me an alcoholic and threatening divorce. This was the last thing I needed. I felt that I couldn't do anything right, that I wasn't good enough. I wanted to feel important, appreciated, and loved. My wife's reaction to my drinking and withdrawal was a painful insult and simply fueled a more intense spiral of drinking so as to escape the pain of the degrading comments. In our own minds, we were both justified in our responses to each other, but those responses only made our problems worse.

Another painful thread in this unraveling was my relationship with my stepson, Adam, which worsened with a difficult situation that arose in 2017. Adam had a high school sweetheart, Emily. They're a great couple, and we all like Emily very much. She comes from a religious family that lives nearby, and she shares our values. But Emily became pregnant in 2016 with our grandson, Isaiah, when she and Adam were seventeen and unmarried.

Tina and I were extremely disappointed in Adam. Adam is one of the smartest kids I've ever known, and I thought he had a bright future that included studying at an elite university. He was planning to pursue mechanical engineering. I assumed that having a baby would prevent any of those plans from coming to fruition. I also believed in the traditional order—marriage first, then kids—so I took the development as a reflection of a moral failure that was shared by the whole family. I supposed that I hadn't done my job as a father very well. Tina and I understood how difficult it would be for them to form a stable family at their age. And of course, we were also aware of the talking that would go on in our community. At times like this, the closeness and caring of a small community is a double-edged sword.

We were upset about it for months. Tina cried a lot, while I dove deeper into alcohol and tobacco. I asked God why this had to happen to our family. Once again, I was in uncharted territory. The situation would have been difficult for anyone, but my reaction didn't help. Our anger and judgmentalism weren't the right approach.

Adam did what probably every seventeen-year-old would do. He panicked and got angry with himself. What he needed at that point was support and love rather than condemnation, but I couldn't see that in the emotions at the time. We had ugly confrontations.

With the calm of hindsight, I have to admit that Adam and Emily handled it very well. I asked them awkward questions: Are you keeping this child? Or are you putting him or her up for adoption, since you're both so young? Or are you planning to abort this unborn, innocent child? Emily wiped her eyes and replied definitely that they were raising this child. That is when Emily instantly gained our love and support. We started down a more productive path in our interactions with our son and the mother of his child.

Isaiah is now four years old, and Adam and Emily are engaged to be married next year. We couldn't be happier for them.

A Cry for Help

At the time, however, Adam's challenges added another layer to the tension between Tina and me, and another weight on the burden I was carrying on my shoulders. Our household was not a pleasant place to be during that period!

God was waiting patiently for our family to ask for his help, and I was not forgotten by him. I know now that God was there in the midst of my pain. He was looking with caring eyes on my family.

Though I'm embarrassed to admit it, if I'm honest, I must confess that I was at this time lukewarm in my faith. We went to church, but not as regularly as we should have gone. I still prayed frequently, but it was rote, and my heart wasn't in it. I was simply going through the motions. It's a common problem that most people of faith have experienced, but that doesn't make it any more acceptable. In God's mercy, he finds a way to pull us out of these ruts, and he certainly did so with me.

My heart began to be softened about the time that we were dealing with Adam and Emily's situation. The physical, emotional, and spiritual stress came to a head one night when I was in the shop late, listening to a sports broadcast. I felt the weight had become too heavy to bear. I did what I should have done long before: I took it to Jesus.

I have a picture of Jesus in a frame on the east wall of my shop, above the workbench that the boys helped me build. I bought the picture at an auction that was held to sell the things of a friend of mine. Adrian had been through a lot. His father and sister had been murdered by people looking for money for their drug addiction. I helped him through those terrible losses by listening to him pour out his troubles. I spent many late nights in the shop talking with him over the phone, and we cried a lot of tears trying to figure out why it happened. Just as my dad is my idol, Adrian's dad was his. Just as I love my amazing sisters, Adrian loved his as well.

So that picture was a reminder that Jesus is there as a comforter in our darkest times. The time was dark for me. That night, something came over me. I fell down on my knees in front of the image of my Savior and I prayed.

"I can't take this anymore, Lord. I'm done. I don't know what to do."

I didn't believe in divorce. I was Catholic. I had the example of my parents. They were together, through thick and thin, for fifty years. How could I fail to live up to that standard?

"I give up. I completely put myself in your hands. Whatever you want me to do, I'll do it."

I recognized my weakness and had come to the right place for help, but I didn't yet know what the answer to my problems was. I wasn't ready for the profound change that was coming. God knew when I would be ready.

Things at home continued to be bad, but we kept plugging away at life. The kids got involved in sports. During soccer season, the younger boys started playing in a youth league twice a week. During basketball season, they played in a Sunday league, and I also took Troy and Clay to high school games virtually every weekend to watch our neighbor Cole play. Like me, Troy and Clay really enjoyed basketball.

But sports did not bring our family together as a whole. Tina and Adam didn't care for basketball. Tina was never a sports fan of any kind, so she always stayed home or went to visit her mom and dad while we went to games. She had never been allowed to play any sports growing up because her parents didn't have the time to drive her to and from activities. So, she never developed an interest in, or enthusiasm for, athletics.

Even so, we found common family activities to enjoy. Although we didn't practice our Catholic faith as devoutly as we should have, the Church did sometimes provide an opportunity for bonding time. We would often go to Mass together as a family on Sunday mornings. Afterward, if the boys had been good in church, we'd go out to a local restaurant or bowling alley as a reward. Needless to say, with three young boys, those "reward times" were few and far between!

Avoiding the Problems

That is how things stood as the summer of 2017 passed. There were problems at home, but yes, there was no crisis that demanded my immediate attention. There were issues in my soul, but I had learned to suppress the promptings of the Spirit and press on with daily tasks. Life wasn't terrible, but it wasn't great either. God wanted more out of me and wanted to give me greater happiness, but I didn't know it yet.

Earlier that year, my friend Chuck and his wife, Kalyn, bought a house near ours. The house needed some renovation. Chuck knew that I had done some construction work over the years, so he invited me to help out. I was happy for the opportunity to assist Chuck and Kalyn. In honesty, though, I saw more than an opportunity to be kind to friends. I was also relieved to have an excuse to stay away from my own home, which needed spiritual renovation that went beyond my do it yourself skills.

So, I settled into a pattern that summer that was good for getting work done, but bad for my personal life. I would put in eight or nine hours a day at my architectural job, run home to change clothes and grab a bite to eat—usually without the rest of the family—and then go to Chuck's house to work until bedtime.

That was my life for several months leading up to "the day that changed my life." My days of avoiding my problems were numbered. My overworking, oversmoking, and overdrinking were about to come to an abrupt halt.

Chapter 3

THE DAY THAT CHANGED MY LIFE

Any impartial observer could have predicted that I was headed for a reckoning. My family background indicated susceptibility to health problems. My grandmother survived into her nineties, but overcame multiple strokes and bouts with cancer along the way. My uncle Dan survived prostate cancer; my aunt Evelyn survived breast cancer; my uncle Lester died from colon cancer; and another aunt, Doris, died of pancreatic cancer. I had witnessed the devastating impact of cancer and I feared it.

I had done little to improve my chances against my genetic dispositions. By 2017, I had been smoking cigarettes for twenty-six years. I tried nicotine patches and gums and every other method: in all, nine attempts to quit, and no success. To this was added the stress that I've already described, and the drinking that I adopted to deal with all of it. My body was under assault on many fronts.

A "Routine" Surgery

One Saturday morning in late August of 2017, I went outside early to fix a broken tile in our yard. After digging for a while, I felt the need to go to the restroom, so I went inside to sit on the toilet. All that came out was blood. Needless to say, I was concerned, but I was too busy to deal with it at that point. I went back to work in the yard.

The boys had soccer games that morning, so I took a break for a few hours to attend those. When I returned home, I went back to digging. I made another trip to the restroom and this time, it was even worse. I was committed to going to Chuck's place to help on his house later that day, so I put my concerns aside. I did tell Tina what had happened and, as expected—and as was completely understandable—she was worried. She insisted I go to the doctor. Like many guys, I avoided the doctor's office as much as I could. I didn't want to admit that I needed help. I didn't like people poking around at my body. I didn't want to spend the money. But I knew Tina was right in this case and that I had to give in. On Monday, I called our family physician and went to see him. The bleeding had stopped by that time, but he recommended that I get a colonoscopy.

Later the next week, I had an appointment with a surgeon at our local hospital for the colonoscopy. When

I returned for the follow-up visit, Dr. Kay explained that he had removed some polyps, but everything else was normal. No cancer! I was relieved.

There was a minor problem, though. A large polyp remained in my colon and I would need surgery to remove it. I asked him if it was anything to worry about, and he assured me it wasn't. It was not cancerous. But there was a possibility it could develop into cancer, and considering my family history, the odds were against me. Dr. Kay said that the surgery was simple, no big deal. It would be over in about twenty minutes. He had done many of them. So, I agreed to have the operation.

I had a deadline at work that I wanted to meet before dealing with the surgery, so we scheduled it for three weeks out. On September 28, 2017, I arrived at the hospital for my polyp removal. The procedure was to start at two in the afternoon and was anticipated to only take about twenty minutes. It wasn't expected to be anything serious and my mother was available to accompany me, so Tina didn't even take off work.

After Dr. Kay cut the polyp out, I was sent to a recovery room. I didn't feel well, and I told the nurses so. They assured me it was nothing to worry about. It was normal not to feel one hundred percent after the surgery.

Still, they insisted, it was necessary for me to eat something before I could be discharged. So, they brought in some food. I tried, but I just couldn't get it down. I began to feel worse. I regurgitated the small amount of food that I had ingested. I knew that was a red flag and the nurses saw it the same way. So much for my quick and easy procedure. I needed to stay overnight for further observation.

That evening, the nurse got me out of bed to take a walk. I felt terrible. After I laid back down, the nurses checked on me, but said little. I didn't understand what was going on. What had happened to my simple, minor operation? I tried to calm myself and get some sleep.

The next day, it was more of the same. Dr. Kay came in to check on me. I was still feeling horrible and told him so. He tried to encourage me: "Ron, we want to get you home." He wanted me to eat. I tried, but after breakfast, I threw up.

This cycle continued to repeat itself over several days. I was supposed to keep walking regularly, but it became increasingly difficult. This was uncharacteristic for me. I'm a hyperactive person, always on the move. When I'd had back surgery several years earlier, I was up and walking afterward—even more than the doctor recommended. So, I was very concerned that my ability to walk was declining and that I kept feeling worse and worse.

I remember various visitors telling me that I was as white as a hospital bed sheet. One told me that I actually looked like I was dead. I was starting to feel that way.

A Second Surgery

On day eight, the sickness was worse than ever. Finally, Dr. Kay decided something had to be done. I was taken into emergency surgery and opened up again. I was cut from my sternum to just below my waist.

It came as no surprise to me when I heard the report that something was in fact wrong. During the first operation, the surgeon incorrectly performed surgery on my intestines. The wound allowed the contents of my colon to leak into my abdominal cavity, causing a severe infection.

After the surgery, Tina, Adam, Emily, Troy, and Clay came to the hospital to see me. I remember looking at them as they sat in my room, unable to see them clearly. Their faces looked like they were melting, or like a painting with water running over it. This disability in my sight was my first clue that something was still seriously wrong with my situation. I started to wonder if their distorted faces were going to be my final memory of them.

Tina stayed by my side in the hospital throughout the day. My parents, brothers, sisters, and sister-in-law had been in the waiting room during the surgery and then visited me later in the day. The recovery from surgery did not go as planned. Massive bleeding continued. My legs started turning blue and my feet began tingling from the swelling caused by the surgeries, a sign that circulation to them was shutting down.

When that happened, I immediately thought of my nephew Caleb, who had been paralyzed in the tragic car accident. I saw what Caleb had gone through with his injuries and I was terrified. I didn't tell anyone that, because I didn't want to upset them by falsely suggesting that my situation was somehow comparable to his. I hated the fact that I understood some of what he was going through every day.

While this medical crisis was in full swing, I received an important visitor. Father Alex was a newly ordained priest who was serving as parochial vicar at our parish. He was making one of his regular visits to the hospital to minister to Catholics and anyone in need. I could hear him talking with a nurse.

"Is there anybody in trouble or discomfort?" he asked.

The nurse replied, "Ron here is in a lot of trouble."

The young priest entered my room.

"Ron, I understand you're in some trouble," he began.

"Father, I'm going to die today." I was scared and souped up on drugs, but I said it matter-of-factly, because I was convinced of the truth of that statement. I was certain that my time was up.

Father Alex remained calm. Priests are trained to deal with these situations. Father Alex was new to the ministry, but over the course of his life, he would probably accompany hundreds of parishioners as they neared death.

"Would you like to confess your sins?" he asked.

"Yes, I would."

For Catholics, the prayers offered in serious illness or at the time of death are considered a sacrament, the anointing of the sick. The rite includes the opportunity to confess your sins, to come clean about your faults as you prepare to meet your Maker.

Father Alex pulled the curtain around the bed to create a semblance of privacy. I began my confession. I mentioned two or three sins and then started crying uncontrollably. The reality of what was happening confronted me. My last rites.

Father finished the prayers and did his best to encourage me.

"I hope everything gets better and you get healthy, Ron."

I knew better. "Father, I am going to die today."

"Be strong. Follow God," he replied sympathetically, and then he left.

Shortly after Father's visit, Tina and the nurses came back into my room. There was blood everywhere. My legs just kept getting bluer. Tina could tell my spirits were sinking. She asked, "What do you want me to do?"

That's when I told her, "Tina, you gotta get me out of here. I'm gonna die."

A Rough Ride

My cousin is married to a doctor who works in the same hospital, and Tina had his number in her phone. She called him and explained my situation. He told her that I was in serious trouble and that she should come down to his floor and talk to him. "Don't take the elevator," he said. "Run."

She did. Breathless after her run down the stairs, she exchanged information with the doctor, and he concluded that I needed to be transferred. "Get him out of here, now," he urged; he told her to transfer me to an urban hospital about an hour away. They quickly filled out the discharge papers.

While the process of transferring me to another hospital was in the works, Tina learned some news that intensified her fears. (I was told about it later.) I had texted one of my best friends, Jake, telling him I needed help. It was a Friday night. High school football is a big deal in our area, and our town's team was playing one of its conference rivals. Jake was at the game. He texted me back asking me what I needed and wondering if it could wait until after the game. He had visited me a few times in the hospital and knew I wasn't doing well. But he didn't know just how serious my condition had gotten. I told him I needed him now. So, he left the game instantly and came over. He saw that I was in terrible shape. He pulled Tina outside the room and told her about an older lady on whom Dr. Kay had performed a similar surgery a few weeks prior to mine. She had not recovered and ended up dying a short time later.

By this time, I was in and out of consciousness, pummeled by the one-two punches of pain and drugs. When I arrived at the ground floor in preparation for exiting the hospital, I became aware of nurses and doctors gathered behind me over my left shoulder in conversation. They were discussing how to transport me to the other hospital, which was about seventy miles away. A CareFlight by helicopter would take about two hours—one hour to get to my hospital and then an hour return trip. The other option was a medevac van, which would take roughly ninety minutes. I heard the concluding remark: "He doesn't have an extra half hour." I would be going by van. Tina would drive separately behind the medevac.

I remember them changing my bandages as they prepared me for transport. The amount of blood I was losing was unbelievable. My stomach was still open from the surgery. They loaded me into the dark blue medevac vehicle. My feet were toward the doors. The ride was so uncomfortable I couldn't bear it. There was a nurse or some other medical professional in the corner of the cargo area. I was weeping and I kept looking over at the man, saying, "Please help me. I'm gonna die. Please help me."

The Vision

We were about twenty minutes down the road when a figure appeared to my left. It was a man, visible from the sternum up, dressed in an off-white robe. He was wearing dark, wraparound sunglasses, and his hair was brown, merging into sandy blond, and brushed upward. I directed one of my pleas toward him: "Please help me, I'm gonna die." Then I blacked out.

When I next awoke, we had arrived at the emergency room. I suppose it's my architecture training, but I remember vividly the appearance of the reception counter, a half-height wall that teed into the main wall on the left side. Across the counter, I glimpsed the receptionist, and once again I voiced my pitiful call for help: "Please help me, I'm gonna die." At that point, I felt that I was truly on the verge of death.

Again, the mysterious figure appeared over my left foot. He had the same face, no sunglasses on, and was wearing the same robe. But now, his hair was down, and it seemed darker on his head and lighter and curlier toward the lower ends just below his shoulders. Now I could see his face more clearly. His eyes were hazel, his face was darkened by five o'clock shadow, and he had a split chin. I noticed that his robe was torn around his neck, the hole just large enough to get his head through.

I implored him, "Please help me. Please give me a second chance."

After I'd uttered my plea to the fellow on the left, I noticed other figures farther to my right. It was a group of six. Like the man on the left, I could only see them from their sternums up. I recognized four of them instantly. My nephew Caleb was directly to the man's left, along with his younger brother Connor. Next to them were two of my sons, Troy and Clay. The other two were a mystery to me. One I could see clearly: a beautiful little girl—two years old, I guessed—with blond curly hair. Beside her was an adult male with gray hair, placed behind the others. His face was somewhat blurred. I recognized neither the girl nor the older man, who was about my age.

As I took in the scene, I couldn't believe my eyes. But I was in no position to question or analyze. My eyes moved back to the person I had decided was Jesus.

I begged him again, "Please, please, give me a second chance."

He didn't reply, but he nodded his head. As soon as he nodded his head, I felt a rush of comfort. At that time, I knew that I was going to be alright.

As soon as a physician approached me, all of these figures disappeared. The surgeon put his hands on my shoulders. "Mr. Schoen," he said, "You're going to be fine. I've gotcha."

Then everything went black again.

The ICU

When I woke up, I had never been in so much pain in my life. I'd begun the second stage in the fight for my life—the ICU—which lasted for ten days.

It was October 7, 2017, nine days after I'd first entered the hospital for my "routine" surgery. I had been transported to the trauma center at a major urban hospital, at the entryway of which I had the extraordinary vision described above. It was the finest emergency care in west central Ohio, so I was in good hands. I was evidently in and out of consciousness and lost track of time, but I'm told that I was kept overnight and then taken into my second emergency surgery the following day.

I remember my mouth being extremely dry and asking for a drink of water or apple juice. I don't know why I asked for apple juice, since I'm not even a big fan of it. But you get strange cravings in these situations. In my condition, they couldn't give me either, though, so they gave me a moist swab. It wasn't enough. The thirst and discomfort were hard to bear, but the pain was worse. I cannot imagine anyone putting up with that much pain for that long. I certainly struggled with it. At one point, I reached my right hand over to my left arm to rip off the skin in a desperate attempt to try to distract myself from the pain in the rest of my body. The pain was a thousand times worse than any I'd ever experienced before. I was allowed to push my button every fourteen minutes for pain meds, and I couldn't push it often enough. I had seven colorful bags of meds hooked up to me at one time. The medication was inadequate; the pain remained unbearable.

At this point in time, I knew that I could live through this crisis physically. But I was asking myself if I wanted to because I didn't think I could take it much longer. There's no doubt in my mind that God took over and got me through it. I'd always been told that God only allows you to handle as much pain as you can take before He takes over. I believe that, but I also believe that He sometimes lets you go right to the limit!

In the midst of the agony, I remember asking my nurses for my phone. I have a picture of my nephew Caleb, along with his brothers, Cameron and Connor, as my screen saver. Just seeing his picture gave me the strength to continue fighting. I told myself that if he could fight through his many, many surgeries, not to mention all of the challenges that followed, I needed to do so as well. I was learning, through the fires of suffering, to identify with the weaknesses and troubles of others.

After a couple of days in ICU, I finally got some water. It was progress! And a great relief to return moisture to my parched mouth. The nurses were still in my room every half hour, checking on me and monitoring vital signs, because I wasn't "out of the woods" yet. My mind was mushy—from pain or meds or a combination of both. I remember a male nurse constantly asking me which hospital I was at. I couldn't tell him. I didn't know. My family would come and see me daily. My brother Steve was especially conscientious in repeating where I was, but I'd forget instantly.

I also remember the male nurses coming in and transferring me to a new bed every day. In retrospect, I'm surprised they needed so much muscle to do the job. When this whole thing started, I weighed 192 pounds. But by the time I exited the ICU, I'd lost forty-seven of those. To say that I was weak is an understatement.

The misery of the ICU dragged on. I hardly slept. When the excruciating pain in my stomach wasn't keeping me from rest, it was the noise of the CareFlight helicopter flying in and out of the hospital throughout the night. One of the nurses told me that most of the activity was related to drug overdoses and auto accidents. I realized that I wasn't the only suffering person in the world.

I do have a positive memory from this period. One of my nephews, Evan, came to visit me almost every Friday on his way home from college. He has no idea how much that meant to me. I looked forward to seeing him every week. Evan and his twin brother, Alex, came into this world roughly two and a half months earlier than expected, but they grew up healthy and strong. They both joined the Army, as well as their younger brother, and the twins are now in the National Guard. I remember Evan sitting in the chair at the right side of my bed. Whenever it was time to move me to another bed for cleaning the sheets (and me), he popped out of his chair, ready and willing to help. I remember telling the nurse that he could help move me; that I trusted him entirely. Of course, they couldn't permit him to help because of hospital regulations, but the fact that he offered and wanted to help however he could will forever be ingrained in my memory.

The Miracle Man

At last, ten days after my second emergency surgery, it was my day of promotion. I was transferred out of ICU! I would have my own single room. As the nurses were rolling me up to my room on the third floor, we encountered the doctor who had met and reassured me at the hospital entry and who had performed the reparative emergency surgery that saved my life. He was accompanied by a retinue of physician interns and other trainees. When he saw me, he stopped and announced, "Hey, everybody, here's 'Miracle Man,' the guy I was telling you about. He tried to 'check out early,' but now he's beating what he wasn't supposed to beat." He started clapping. Then his team followed suit, applauding and whistling. I started crying my eyes out. He put his hands on my shoulders, bent down to me, whispered into my right ear, "I told you I had you," and gently hugged my upper chest.

I wept during the entire remainder of my journey to my new room. All along the way, hospital staff and others smiled, said, "good job" and clapped their hands. I was brimming with gratitude toward my surgeon and all of the outstanding staff who had brought me back from the verge of death. I was overwhelmed with gratitude toward God. He had heard my pleas. He had given me the second chance that I'd begged for.

Chapter 4

THE RECOVERY

I was out of mortal danger, but that didn't mean my life suddenly got easy. I needed a massive amount of physical healing, which would only come slowly. I also needed to process emotionally and spiritually what had happened and how I would respond. My second chance was just beginning, and I still had a lot to learn.

Grateful

One thing I learned during my recovery was to be grateful for others. My entire stay at the hospital to which I was transferred was blessed with amazing people: doctors, nurses, cooks, and everyone else. My recuperation was difficult, but it was made bearable by the loving people who surrounded me: family, friends, regular caregivers, and strangers I encountered briefly along the way.

Nurses would come in regularly to check my vitals. Whenever I ran out of whatever fluids were going into me, the machines would loudly BEEP... BEEP... BEEP. They would go on like that until a nurse came in to change the bags. It's a sound similar to the one made by large commercial vehicles backing up, and I still have flashbacks to the hospital experience virtually every time I hear those warning sounds. I consider that beeping to be the worst sound in the world.

My caregivers didn't know this, but there were several nights that I stayed up past midnight working on feet and toe exercises, because I was anxious to speed up the process of recovery. Slowly, but surely, I made progress. October 16 was my forty-fourth birthday. It was hands down my best birthday ever. For one thing, it was the birthday that, for a time, I didn't think I would ever see. For another, as a result of the swelling in my legs decreasing, I was walking better. And finally, the hospital staff once again demonstrated their thoughtfulness and caring by recognizing the day in a special way.

One of the hospital cooks, an older man, brought up a small cake. When he entered the room, seven or eight nurses came with him, singing "Happy Birthday." I went to tears. The cake was a circle of about nine inches in diameter, topped with thick, white frosting and a few candles. Three years later, I still have the picture of it on my phone. I hope I never forget it or accidentally delete it.

Later that evening, some of my coworkers came to visit me. I had just finished eating a meal when the cake had been brought up—not to mention I hadn't gotten approval from my dietician for this sugary delight—so I hadn't eaten any of the cake. Instead, I gave my coworkers some small pieces. They brought me a large "Get Well Soon" card that was signed by the other employees at my firm. That meant more to me than they'll ever know as well. It was the additional fuel I needed to keep going.

Shortly after my coworkers left, my family came to see me. I think Mom and Dad smiled the entire time they were there. They were happy because I was getting my color back and they could see that I was getting better. I had made it to a birthday that, based on my physical condition a few weeks earlier, I should never have reached. My brothers and one of my sisters, Diana, were making their usual jokes trying to cheer me up. Growing up, our family never showed much affection, but we siblings always looked out for one another. That was our way of expressing our love for each other. Mom and Dad never vocalized "I love you" either. But we all knew—and know—that they love us as much as we love them.

The next day, I woke up at my usual time, which was around four o'clock in the morning. Later that morning, my team of doctors came in and did my morning checkup. The team always consisted of one of my lead doctors plus anywhere from four to eight medical students. They would check on the progress of my stomach and ask me questions. A little later that same morning, my dietician came in and told me what I could eat. I asked her if I could eat some of my birthday cake. My coworkers had eaten half of it and left me the remainder. I was so excited. I was ready to dig in! She told me I could only eat a really thin slice.

I obeyed. It was better than nothing, but not by much!

Humor is an indispensable tool in helping you get through health trials, and there were many opportunities for it. Flowers arrived from a friend whom I'd worked with for over twenty years. I called him afterward and joked about how the gift seemed more appropriate for a different outcome: "Thanks for the flowers, but obviously I lived."

Pondering Life

When I didn't have visitors, I had four walls to stare at—all day, every day. There are twenty-four hours in a day, and in a hospital bed, if you get one or two hours of sleep at a time, that's a victory. I spent a lot of time thinking and praying. One thing I stewed about was the cause of my difficulty. I was extremely angry with the doctor who had botched the minor surgery that he said he had performed hundreds of times. I suppose I had a deep sense that complete healing would have a spiritual as well as a physical dimension, and that forgiveness would be part of that process. But, as my physical pain was still too intense to put behind me, dealing with the emotional damage was something that took lower priority. I knew that I had to forgive the doctor like God teaches us. But I wasn't ready for that yet.

One more pleasant matter that occupied my thoughts was trying to interpret the vision I'd had at the hospital reception area. The first thing I needed to know was whether it was real or not. Maybe it had been nothing more than a dream. I thought about the image of the half wall I'd noticed and thought it might be a piece of solid evidence to investigate.

I decided to enlist the assistance of Amy, one of my nurses. There were several nurses who helped me as I tried to recover my ability to walk. Before feeling in my legs returned, I couldn't make it to the restroom. That was hard to deal with, and humiliating. There are so many things that we take for granted in life until they are taken from us. There is a feeling of ignorance and helplessness when you're unable to perform basic functions that had become second nature. Whatever you need to relearn, you appreciate.

Amy was amazing, like an angel. I asked her to help my investigation.

"Amy, is there any chance you could take me to where I was brought into this building?"

She paused, puzzled. "Yeah, probably. Why?"

"I just need to see something." She agreed to humor me.

I wasn't yet strong enough for the stairs, so we took the elevator. During the elevator ride, I had briefly explained what I was looking for. When we reached the ground floor, we got out of the elevator and walked just outside of the ICU, where I stood holding onto the railing. Amy asked if I was ready to see what was on the other side of the door.

I responded, "I don't want to go in, but is there any way you could open one of those doors so I can see in?"

"Sure."

The door opened and there it was. There was a different receptionist, but the counter and half wall were identical to what I had seen before. I was sure of it.

"So, I didn't dream all of this stuff up," I thought to myself.

We returned to my room.

Now I had to figure out what the vision meant. Concerning the man on the left, there was no doubt in my mind that it was Jesus. Of course, I recognized Caleb, Connor, Troy, and Clay. But who was the little girl? I ran through mental images of my nieces and other youngsters I knew; it wasn't any of them. And there was the other guy in the background. I couldn't determine who he was either. I also still wasn't sure why I'd been visited by these figures.

In addition to puzzling over the vision, I reflected on who I was and who I should be. I regretted the dumb things I'd done. And I realized that I had received the second chance that I'd begged for. Teams of doctors and their understudies kept coming in. "This is Ron, the miracle man," was the way I was often introduced. One asked, "Ron, do you understand how lucky you are?" I wasn't feeling well at the time, but I honestly responded, "Yes, I do." The physician replied, "The chance of you surviving that is zero. Nobody survives that." He pointed out that, considering the condition I was in and everything that had to be removed and redone, it was simply incredible that I'd pulled through.

It seemed clear. I had been given a genuine, miraculous, second chance.

A Revelation

My recuperation period also brought a stunning revelation. During the entire episode, I had assumed that the conclusion given me by the initial assessment was accurate, and that there was no cancer, just a large polyp. A little over a week before my release from the hospital, a doctor came in early one morning to check my status and asked if I'd been given my results from the previous day. (Medical tests were being run constantly during this time.) I replied that I had not, but I had been given some the previous day. During the course of the exchange, the doctor got an inkling that my information seemed to be incomplete. As our conversation continued, he said, "Your cancer results came back clear. You do know that you had cancer, correct?"

I was absolutely floored. "Wait a minute. What did you say?" I'm seldom without words, but I had no more at this time.

"You were told you had cancer, right?"

I thought he was mistaken. "No, I wasn't. I had the surgery so it wouldn't turn into cancer."

The doctor came closer and said in a low voice, "Ron, you had cancer."

At first, I was completely dumbfounded. I couldn't believe that no one had told me this. It took me some time to digest the news. I was absolutely devastated.

Three weeks before Thanksgiving, I was discharged from the hospital. I had been under intense medical care for more than a month, but I had made it. I would live. But how would I live? Now I had to put into practice the thoughts and realizations that had come to me during my health crisis. I had begged for a second chance, and I'd been given one. What would I do with it? I'd been struggling—hard—for weeks to keep on living. I had recovered a large part of my physical strength. Now I needed to figure out the spiritual meaning of my experience. Now I needed to find God's will for my life.

Chapter 5

LIVING MY SECOND CHANCE

Being discharged from the hospital did not mean that my health challenges had disappeared. I would need to develop a whole new routine to deal with my new situation. I would also continue to struggle to understand and assimilate my experience, including the mysterious vision. Even as I strove to reform my life to make the most of my second chance, I still fought against old temptations and long-simmering problems. How could I forgive the person whose mistake had sent me into this physical tailspin? How could I become a better husband and father and build the happy family life that I envisioned? These struggles are far from over. Some of them, I admit, may go on as long as I draw breath. But that doesn't mean that I couldn't make the most of my second chance. I was determined to do so.

A New Routine

From the hospital, I was sent to a nursing home for ten days to live and get the therapy that I needed to build my strength back up. Fortunately, I was transferred to a nursing home in my hometown. My youngest sister, Diana, worked there at the time. She came in every morning before starting her shift to check on me and see if I needed anything. She would also take my dirty clothes home and wash them for me every other day. She was such a blessing to me through that period.

Another true blessing while I was living at the nursing home was an old neighbor who I grew up down the road from. His name was Dan. Dan would come to the nursing home almost daily to visit and pray with and for his dad, Don. When I was growing up, Don hired me in the summer to help him clean his chicken coop out. Unfortunately, Don had a stroke quite a few years ago, which has confined him to a wheelchair. So, one day, I was resting in my room after therapy when Dan wheeled his dad into my room. He asked me if I wanted to say part of the Rosary with him and Don. I said, "yes, I'd really enjoy that, but I don't have my Rosary with me." He said "here, I always bring an extra one with me." So, Dan and I said part of the Rosary as his dad, Don, listened. Dan has since finished his training, and is now a deacon.

During the day, I did therapy to get my strength back in my legs by walking and climbing stairs. I also did other exercises to build my upper body strength back up so that I could take care of myself at home. I knew that Tina would need to be at work and our three boys would be in school, so I wanted to be as self-reliant as possible.

But that self-reliance wouldn't be immediate. The damage done to my excretory system meant that I needed an ileostomy to deal with my body's waste. When the surgeons at the second hospital performed the emergency surgery, they cut a four-inch diameter hole into my stomach, which is where the stool went while the remainder of my colon healed. The bag was attached to the right side of my stomach. The surgeries also left a lot of stitches running from my sternum to my waist. My healing would take time, and I couldn't do it alone.

After the ten-day stay at the nursing home, I finally returned to my family. My daily routine was to be dramatically different from what it had been before my adventure began in September. Previously, Tina and I—like most people—had a typical schedule. Tina's alarm went off at 4:00 a.m., and she was out the door to work around 5:10. I got to sleep in; my alarm didn't go off until 5:30 a.m. I'd get ready for work, get the boys prepared for school, and then leave for my architecture job.

In the new routine, my days began with rolling out of bed to dump my ileostomy bag. Sometimes, I needed to do it once or twice during the night. Occasionally, I needed Tina's help, but I usually tried not to wake her, so I'd attempt it on my own by rolling out of bed and then slowly getting to my feet. Sometimes, I slipped off the side of the bed and fell onto the floor, and had to get up from there. After Tina was off to work, my alarm would go off to prompt me to get the boys up for school. I was their alarm, yelling until they got out of bed. There were many days the boys would come into my bedroom and help me get out of bed. The three of them would take turns doing this. I struggled to get up on my own because all of my stomach muscles were cut. This was yet another thing I took for granted in life until I lost it.

When the boys left for school, I was on my own for a couple of hours. I have two aunts, Dian and Ethel, who are retired nurses, and they generously agreed to take turns coming to help. One or the other came every morning during the week to change my dressings and empty the ileostomy bag. My mother would also come to assist, and nurses from the hospital occasionally checked in and changed some dressings in the afternoons. Other family members and friends would chip in when the others weren't available. My oldest brother, Chris, and even Adam's fiancée, Emily, came over and handled the job once. On the weekends, it was usually my neighbor Beth, who is also a nurse.

Naturally, I had a number of medical appointments during my recovery. When I wasn't allowed to drive yet, other people would transport me. One of my classmates from school, Karen, helped once, as did my youngest brother, Ken. The majority of the time, my oldest brother, Chris, would drop what he was doing and drive.

All of these people offered to help before I even had a chance to ask. Their generosity reminded me of how blessed I truly am. I experienced the love of God through the charity of these good people.

I remember my two aunts and my mom "arguing" in a good-natured manner over who would get to help me each day. I think what I enjoyed the most about their visits was the time we would spend after the health care tasks were over. They usually stayed a little while and talked. The fact that they dropped everything they were doing in their daily life to spend a few hours to physically help me, and more importantly, to see how I was doing mentally, will never be forgotten. There were several days that my aunt Ethel and I would drink coffee and lose track of the time. There were times that I'd run out of bandages and Dian would go and get more. And my parents … well, I can't properly put into words how much they have been there for me. My dad usually drove Mom to my house to change my dressing, and she always brought a plate of cookies. Dad would usually start off watching some TV, then take a quick nap. To this day, my mom is extremely worried and overprotective of me, and as a parent, I get it.

After everyone left, I usually spent as much time as possible walking around my house, trying to build my strength more. But I still found myself all alone for hours, looking at four walls and talking to God. I reflected on how thankful I was for a lot of people and a lot of things. Surprisingly, one of the things that I was thankful for was getting cancer. Don't get me wrong, I do not believe that cancer is a gift from God. But I began to feel grateful that I was the one who got it and had to go through everything, rather than my family or friends having to suffer that way. I will also be forever grateful to God for giving me the strength to defeat this horrible disease. I am grateful for everything that I encountered along the way—for the way the experience changed me. And finally, I am grateful to God for sending all of the doctors, nurses, family members, and everyone else who became a blessing during that time.

A New Outlook

As I continued to recuperate, I also continued to reflect on my experience and what it meant for me. One thing I couldn't get out of my mind was the vision—in particular, the mystery of who the two unidentified figures were. The other figures in the image I saw seemed to be people who God had used or was using to help me in some way. Were the others also important people on my journey to making the most of my second chance, to growing closer to God, and to becoming a better person?

As I sought an answer to that question, I began to establish a different way of life. One improvement was giving up my addictions. I admit that this was more a health necessity than a virtuous decision, but either way, it was an important step in the right direction. I stopped smoking the day before my first surgery, and

I haven't smoked since. After so many tries, I've finally kicked the habit! I drink a few beers occasionally, but I no longer abuse alcohol as I did before. Clean living is beneficial to physical, financial, and spiritual health. I hope I have the grace never to fall into those habits again.

I had always wanted to do a Bible study, but never had the opportunity or never got around to it. Shortly before my health crisis, Dave, a friend of mine who lives down the road who used to play softball with me, asked if I wanted to join him and a few other guys to start a Bible study at his home. I told him that I always wanted to do this, but I was embarrassed to admit that I'd never read a Bible before. I had tried many times when I was younger, but just couldn't understand it or stay interested enough to persevere. Dave told me it didn't matter; there were a few others who had never read the Bible either. So, I eagerly agreed to attend.

About two weeks before the first scheduled session, I had my "routine" surgery. My participation in the study never happened, and they went on without me. Dave told me later that the group prayed for me every time they met, which was once a week. When they began a second cycle of study the following year, I finally got to join. Although I had grown up Catholic, reading the Bible wasn't something my family had done. So, I was intimidated by the prospect of reading the Word of God by myself. The best thing about this study group is that it made me more comfortable about opening up and reading scripture on my own. Now, I subscribe to a Catholic scripture magazine and read from it almost every day.

We studied the Bible for about a year. At this time, the group is on hiatus because several of the families involved are expecting babies. But we hope to resume soon. I love to study God's Word with other people, to become more aware of His presence in the world and to grow in my relationship with fellow Christians.

Another motivation for plunging deeply into God's Word was a new friend who also helped me solve part of the mystery of my vision.

A New Friend

A few weeks after I'd come home from the hospital, the doorbell rang. It was an acquaintance of mine, Scott. We had first met about fifteen years earlier, when we were competing to purchase the same house. (He won.) I would see him every so often, but I never knew him well.

I invited him inside, and he entered with a bottle of cinnamon schnapps. I told him to have a seat and asked why he'd brought the schnapps. "Whenever you're feeling better, you can sip on this," he replied." I didn't really drink liquor and was a little puzzled by the visit and the gift, but I appreciated the gesture.

We ended up talking for half an hour. I began to discover what a terrific person Scott is. Over the course of our conversation, he asked how my ordeal had started, and I explained that it was a colon exam. I described my situation a bit more, and then the conversation moved on. As we bid each other goodbye, I looked forward to getting to know Scott better.

A week or two later, I saw Scott's wife, Jenny, after church. She asked me how I was doing and then thanked me for telling Scott about the symptoms I had experienced leading up to my colon trouble.

"You're welcome," I replied.

"You don't understand," she said meaningfully.

I looked at her, confused. "You're right. I don't."

"Scott's had the same symptoms."

"Oh no," I thought.

When Scott went in for his colon exam, it revealed that he had stage 4 colon cancer. Ever since, Scott has been in the fight of his life. During the course of his chemotherapy and radiation treatments, the doctors discovered that the cancer had spread to his liver as well.

About six months after I'd returned home, I decided to check in on Scott. I texted him and offered to chat. I would bring the donuts and he would provide the coffee. We spent an hour on Saturday morning at his dining room table, just talking about life. A couple of weeks later, we did it again. A connection was starting to form in my mind. Three weeks later, we met again. The idea started to sink in. I decided to vocalize it.

"Scott, you aren't gonna believe this, but I'm pretty sure I saw you during my trouble." I had come to believe that he was the unknown, gray-haired figure in my vision.

I told him the whole story. He just stared at me. He didn't know what to say. I admitted that I wasn't a hundred percent sure—the face in the vision wasn't clear—but I was pretty sure because of the shade of gray color, the way it was parted, and the shape of his head. I asked him if he thought I was crazy. "No, not at all. I have a hard time believing that someone would or even could make something like that up," was his reply.

One half of the mystery from my vision had been solved.

After a lot of additional chemo and radiation, Scott's doctors decided to cut as much of the cancer out of his liver as was safely possible. I joked with him about the similarities of our health challenges: "Wow, you're really competitive." He had to get cut from his sternum down to his stomach like I did, except his went over to his side. So, he has a large "L" carved across his front torso—which in our little world obviously stands for "Lucky," because he made it through the surgery. Scott has continued to go through different types of chemo on and off for roughly the past three years. About a year ago, tests showed the cancer had metastasized. Now, he also has it in his lungs, back and brain.

To this day, Scott and I are good friends. He's still driving a school bus, farming, and being a husband, dad, friend, church communion distributor, and an inspiration to everyone. He's absolutely amazing, and I thank God every day for our friendship.

Recently, I went to see Scott and Jen. I wanted to let him know how much our friendship meant. "You've changed me," I said.

"How?" he replied.

I explained: "I'd never opened the Holy Bible before. You told me you read the Bible every morning. Now, I read it every day."

We've continued to get together regularly for coffee and donuts. My friendship with Scott has been an important part of my life. With God's grace and Scott's example, I've immersed myself in the Word and my outlook on life has changed radically. I am starting to understand why I got a second chance. It forced me to take a huge step back and look at the world and my place in it with new eyes. Just as Scott's face had been blurry in the vision, but was now clear, so my view of the world had been distorted and was now being set. I still had a lot of work to do to share God's view on everything, but at least I knew what my purpose was.

The Blue-Eyed Girl

As I was recovering, I continued to search out the identity of the final figure in my vision. I even brought the matter to my priest, trying to get some perspective on the strange event. I had been on meds, after all, and was in terrible pain. Could it have been a meaningless hallucination? I didn't believe that, but I questioned my own judgment. I thought it might help to have an expert opinion.

When I saw Father Alex, I thanked him for his visit during my rough period in the hospital and then asked him about the vision. He listened carefully while I described it. I asked him if he thought it could be divinely inspired. Or was it just a mental glitch? Was I crazy at the time?

Father Alex said he didn't have enough experience to make an informed judgment, so he referred me to an older priest. I repeated my explanation, and the more experienced pastor concluded that no, I was not crazy. I was relieved! He had worked a great deal in hospital ministry, and he said it was not uncommon for people on the verge of death to have encounters, even conversations, with Jesus. He said he did not question the belief that I had seen Jesus. I saw this priest's approval as confirmation of what I already knew in my heart to be true.

Now, who was that blue-eyed girl?

During my convalescence, I made frequent trips to the pharmacy in Coldwater to pick up my medications. At some point, I noticed a display on the counter of bracelets of various colors. They were emblazoned with the words "Scarlett the Brave."

One day, as the boys were preparing to return to school after a weekend, I went to buy supplies at a store in town. There was a collection jug with the same words: "Scarlett the Brave." I put some money in.

The next time I was in town, I was confronted by a huge sign with, yet again, the intriguing words "Scarlett the Brave." Who was this person, and why was her name constantly being brought to my attention? I didn't yet realize it, but the revelation of the blue-eyed girl's identity was gradually unfolding.

After five months of rest at home, I was finally able to return to work. It was great to get back to the office. I was happy to see everyone. Most of them came to see me at least once at one of the hospitals, the nursing home, or at home when I was recovering. I'm truly blessed to work for, and with, so many great people.

One day, Troy came home from school with two coupons to a local restaurant, a reward for completing a certain amount of reading. Tina and I took Troy and Clay out for dinner that evening. The restaurant had a bar and, after we finished eating, a band started setting up for its gig. It was about seven o'clock. I didn't like to have the kids around with people drinking, so I was anxious to leave. But the boys wanted to stay to shoot baskets and play pool in the game room in the back of the building. So, I agreed to stick around a while longer. The boys took up with another youngster who was playing in the back, the son of one of the band members.

When the band was ready, the lead singer introduced himself at the microphone and announced, "I want everyone to know that all proceeds tonight go to my niece, Scarlett the Brave." Scarlett, he explained, was a two-year-old girl who was battling cancer. My interest was piqued.

The band started playing, and they were very good. I was enthralled. They were selling CDs for one dollar for the cause of Scarlett the Brave, and I decided I had to have one. I went up between songs and asked to purchase a CD. I emptied my wallet and handed over the cash. (I prefer currency to plastic, so I'd gone to an ATM for money just before dinner.) The band member looked at me in surprise. "Do you understand how much you've given me?" he asked.

"I do."

"Thank you!"

In return for the donation, I asked for a favor. "I just want you to relay something to this girl and her parents: I got out of the hospital not long ago. I beat cancer. Let them know it's possible. It's very possible. It's hard, but it can happen."

That was my message. Not eloquent, but from the heart. I was starting to believe there was some special connection between me and "Scarlett the Brave."

When we left the restaurant, the kids wanted to go to McDonald's for ice cream. "There's a problem," I confessed. "I don't have any money."

"Didn't you just get cash from the ATM?" Tina asked.

I explained, "Yes, but after I paid for our meal, I donated the remainder to the man with the CD in order to help that little girl."

All we could do was rush home to listen to that (very valuable) CD.

When we arrived at our house, I immediately popped it into my computer. The disc played the band's first song, the one that had captured my attention. It was a beautiful song about a little girl fighting a terrible disease. I couldn't wait to hear more. But that was it. The CD only contained that one song!

I smiled at God's sense of humor. It was the most expensive song I've ever bought, but I didn't regret the purchase. It had gone for a good cause. Again, it was evident that my outlook on life had changed.

The final piece of the puzzle of the blue-eyed girl was put in place, appropriately enough, through my participation in an event that reflected my newfound commitment to deepening my faith. For a number of years, there has been an annual conference for Catholic men in our area. Saint Michael's parish hall in Fort Loramie is about twenty miles away from my home. It holds seven hundred people, but it fills up every year for this dynamic event. In 2018, a friend invited me to attend, so I went for the first time. The speakers were phenomenal, and it was thrilling to be part of such a large gathering of men who take their faith seriously.

During a break, I went outside to get some fresh air and stretch my legs. There, I encountered a friend I hadn't seen in twenty years.

"Trent, good to see you! How are you doing?"

"I'm good," he replied. "What about you? I heard you went through a lot of things."

"Yeah, I did. I still have some complications, but I feel very fortunate and thankful."

Trent had been a classmate and companion of my younger brother. In high school, he was part of a crowd that drank and partied a lot. To be honest, I was surprised to see him at a Catholic men's conference, and I told him so.

"Trent, you seem a little different."

"Yeah, I finally grew up and found God."

Our conversation continued for a while and got more personal. I told him about my vision. I explained that I still hadn't discovered who the little girl was, but I had been consistently drawn to a girl named Scarlett who was battling cancer.

Trent looked at me with meaning in his eyes. "You know who that is, don't you?"

"No, I obviously don't," I replied. "She's everywhere I turn, but I don't know her."

Trent said, "Her mom is my first cousin."

"Really?" I thought for a moment. "How old is she?"

"She's about three now." The age fit, but I needed to know for sure.

"Trent, could you send me a picture?"

The conference was over. I was sitting at home in my recliner a few days later when my phone beeped. It was the photograph from Trent. I stared at it. Tina noticed my reaction.

"What are you doing?" she queried.

"Trent sent me a picture of a little girl he knows. Her name is Scarlett Unrast."

Tina looked at the phone. "Isn't that the little girl in the vision you told me about?"

"Yes," I said. "That's who it is."

It was the face of the girl in my vision.

The final piece of the puzzle fit. Jesus had visited me in my darkest hour and had given me another chance. He brought along people who were to help me and who, in turn, I was to help through assistance and prayer.

Needless to say, I became very interested in little Scarlett and her fate. I discovered the Facebook page for "Scarlett the Brave," where updates were posted and support expressed. The first post reads: "Welcome to Scarlett Unrast's Support Group. Here is where Scarlett's journey begins. This sweet, blue-eyed girl was recently diagnosed with stage 4 high risk cancer (neuroblastoma). Neuroblastoma is a type of cancer that forms in certain types of nerve tissue. Like with Scarlett's, it frequently starts from one of the adrenal glands."

The post is dated October 9, 2017—three days after my vision.

About a year ago, I met Scarlett and her mother. I got her mom's number through my friend Trent and contacted her out of the blue. To make her more comfortable about meeting a perfect stranger, I suggested that we get together at a public park. When the time for the meeting came, I was both excited and nervous.

What would she think about the crazy story I was about to tell her?

When they came walking up at the park, I discovered an interesting coincidence. To my surprise, my cousin Tony was with them! Scarlett's mom, Lindsay, who is divorced, had started dating my cousin.

I warned Lindsay that what I was about to tell her would sound strange, but I assured her it was in earnest. I recounted the vision and everything that had happened since then to bring Scarlett to my attention. I told her I was sure that Scarlett was the girl in my vision. Lindsay was at first skeptical, but as I went on, she came around. She said that she could see the sincerity in my eyes. She recognized that there's no way I would be making up such a story.

It was a relief and a pleasure to finally meet Scarlett and her family and share my experience. We parted on friendly terms, and our paths have crossed a few times since that day. I don't know whether God has yet revealed in its entirety the reason Scarlett was brought into my life, but I am convinced that He did bring us together for a reason. I have been inspired by her story, and I know I'm supposed to continue to pray for and encourage her. I'll never forget her part in the day that changed my life.

Chapter 6

CALLED TO ACTION

I would have always said that I believe in God. But saying is one thing and doing is another. When I was given my second chance, I became convinced that God is real. That is to say, His existence makes a difference. Now, I don't just say that God exists; my actions testify to my belief.

A Changed Man

There are countless ways that my daily life has improved since that life-changing experience in the hospital. I've already mentioned my commitment to reading Scripture. Another habit I've taken on may seem insignificant and mundane, but I assure you it makes a big difference. I've been doing it frequently since this experience, and I'd like to challenge readers to do the same.

Buy someone's meal.

When I'm out, I sometimes try to pay for people's meals without them knowing. Usually, I seek out someone who is elderly, handicapped, or in the military. It's a practice I actually started before my health crisis, but I have since doubled down and expanded it.

One Sunday, after Mass, our family went out for brunch. I noticed an elderly man sitting by himself. I didn't recognize him, but I knew he was the one I should help. After my wife, my kids, and I finished eating, I went to pay for our food. I told the waitress I would cover the elderly gentleman's as well. She said, "Oh, do you know him? That's nice." I explained that I didn't know him at all. She said she would let him know. I replied, "No, please don't tell him until after we leave, or at all." She asked why I was doing it and I said, "Why not?" She smiled.

As we were pulling out of the parking lot in our car, the man came out of the restaurant and caught sight of us. He waved and mouthed the words, "Thank you." I could see tears running down his face. You can imagine the feeling I had from being able to remind someone that they're not alone in life. Even more, God cares. I believe that He is inspiring me to help particular people in this way. All I have to do is be open to the prompting of the Holy Spirit.

On another occasion, Tina and I went to Chicago with my buddy Jake and his wife. We stopped at a Bob Evans on the way. Once again, God tapped me on the shoulder. I scanned the room and then I noticed her.

An elderly lady with some kind of disability in her arm was sitting by herself, about twenty feet away from us. While we were eating, I noticed that the woman struggled to feed herself with her disabled arm. I also noticed that she received a second meal, this one to go. When we were finished, I dashed up to pay our (and her) bill. I asked the cashier not to tell the lady that I paid until after we were gone, but she either misunderstood or ignored me. While we were still in the restaurant, the lady approached the counter; the cashier pointed at me and told her what I'd done, and the woman immediately started crying.

As we left, I kept an eye out for her. I saw her get into an old van parked in a handicapped spot. As she drove by to exit, I saw that there was a man in the passenger seat. I assumed that the passenger was a friend or relative—husband, perhaps—who wasn't healthy enough to go into the restaurant. I understood why God had prompted me to help the lady that day.

Another practice I've adopted is buying meal cards or gas cards and giving them to people who may be in need. I try to find ways of delivering them anonymously. Often, the beneficiaries are people who have cancer or people who need to pay for doctors' visits or therapy bills. This has gotten to be something that I enjoy doing so much that I've asked a few friends to join me. There are now five or six other people who throw in a few dollars—yet another example of how blessed I am to be surrounded by such amazing people.

My final example: The first summer that I got back to work, I began walking at my lunch hour with some coworkers. We would walk around town, roughly two miles. One day, only two of us were available to walk. We were strolling down a nearby alley when I noticed an elderly lady mowing along the canal across the alley from where she lived. She looked very scared of falling in the canal, so I asked her if I could mow a couple rows for her. She said "yes" with a puzzled look on her face. I mowed those rows for her, and then we continued our walk.

Two Saturdays later, I went in to work. As I was finishing up my work for the day, I kept thinking to myself, I wonder if that nice elderly lady needs her lawn mowed. So, I decided to leave work and go over and find out. I drove over, pulled into her lane, and rang her doorbell. She answered the door and I asked her if I could mow her lawn. She looked at me, wondering why. I asked her a second time. Then, she asked me, "How much?" I told her that I didn't want any money and that I just wanted to help her out by mowing her lawn. She finally agreed. So, I mowed her lawn and cleaned her mower deck. Before I left, I asked her if I could come back the next week and mow again. She said, "Well, I suppose that would be OK." The entire drive home I kept wondering why I was drawn to this lady. Why did God choose this lady for me to help? The following Friday, on my way home from work, I stopped in and once again mowed her lawn. She watched me the entire time. I could tell she was wondering the same thing I was, Why is he here? Why is this random guy helping me again? After I finished mowing her lawn, I once again began cleaning her mower deck. As I was cleaning her deck out, I began asking her questions. I really needed to know why God put us together. Well, after a few minutes, I asked her about her husband. Sure enough, there it was … she then told me that she lost her husband to cancer ten years ago after he got out of the military.

The following week, I brought my son Troy with me to help. We mowed, trimmed, and pruned shrubs for a few hours. Rose thanked us, and we went home. On our way home, I asked Troy if he enjoyed himself. He said he did. Then, I asked him if he got "paid." He told me that he didn't understand, and that he didn't get anything. I told him that sometimes in life it isn't the amount of money you get, it's the size of the smile on the person's face that we help.

I mowed Rose's lawn the remainder of the year. Unfortunately, Rose was no longer able to take care of herself and her family put her in a retirement home.

I recommend doing things like these because they're tangible ways of expressing that God is in control through His humble "helping hands." I don't have a lot of money. I drive a 2005 truck. But, as I see it, the money I do have isn't mine, but God's. He's the one telling me to do these things. I don't want it to sound like I'm making a great sacrifice. It can be difficult to give, but the reward is always worth it. The knowledge that I've done what God has asked me to do by assisting someone in need is worth more than the few dollars that I would have otherwise spent on who knows what. Most people have an extra ten or twenty dollars a month that they can part with, if you really think about it. What have you spent it on in the past? Alcohol, tobacco, or potato chips—to name a few—the things I used to spend it on too many times. It's a great feeling to spend it on something far more worthwhile. When you do that, as I see it, it gives you a sense that God's patting you on the back.

I've been the beneficiary of generosity, so I know what it feels like on the other side. The first Christmas that I was home after my hospital stays, my neighbors came over with a box that had a bow on it. I asked them what the box was for. The mother of the family, Karen, explained that every year at Christmas, her immediate family gets together and chooses another family to help. The family members take turns being in charge of selecting the beneficiary family. Karen told me that it was her year to choose, and she chose my family. The box contained a few things that they thought would help us. They told me that even their youngest daughter, Mira, had put something inside. Touched by the gesture, I thanked them, and they left.

When I opened the box, I found "get well" cards, food cards, gas cards, and cash. I instantly got choked up. The cards were helpful and very much appreciated, but what was most poignant were the nickels, dimes, and pennies. Maybe I'm wrong, but I have a feeling little Mira put those in there. There's a lot of good in the world. I've seen it and felt it.

One of the reasons that I decided to write this book is because I've decided to give the profits to families' in need through meals, gas cards, and whatever else God has planned for me to do with it. Because I have complete faith in what God wants me to do, and with your help we can make a few families lives just a little better.

A Work in Progress

I don't want to leave the impression that my life is perfectly in order and canonization as a saint is right around the corner. Far from it! In many ways, the struggles that I was dealing with before I saw Jesus are still there at times.

It was another health issue that brought me face-to-face with one of my biggest spiritual challenges. My stepson, Adam, had some kidney problems, so I went to visit him in the hospital during his treatment. It was around eighteen months after my incident, and I hadn't been back to that hospital since then. I knew all along that I would need to forgive the surgeon who messed up my first two surgeries, but I was still struggling, and still am, to achieve that. At times, I've felt very close to forgiveness. But my hospital visit with Adam showed how far I still had to go.

On the way to see my stepson, I was praying that God would help me handle the situation—that there would be no ugly confrontation with the surgeon. I could tell I wasn't at full forgiveness yet, so my prayer was that I simply wouldn't see Dr. Kay. When I arrived, I walked quickly to the elevator and I visited with Adam, Emily, and our grandson for about an hour. As I left the room, I prayed again that I could escape without seeing Dr. Kay.

I walked past the room where all my trouble had taken place. My nerves were on edge. I continued moving quickly toward the exit. Fifty feet more and I'd be out. Then he walked by.

Anger welled up and I started to shake. Dr. Kay said hello nonchalantly as he passed. Out of the corner of my eye, I saw that, as he went by, he realized who I was. I just continued out the door and to my car. When I got there, I started laughing hysterically. I berated God, in good fun: "Really, you couldn't give me fifty more feet?"

About a year ago, Adam had another kidney complication—and I had another opportunity to test my ability to forgive. I went to pick up Adam from the hospital. I thought that I had made good progress in my spiritual state, and I felt that I was very close to reaching a place of peace and mercy toward Dr. Kay. The medical personnel were rolling Adam out in a wheelchair while I walked along. As we were exiting an elevator, Dr. Kay walked in. I quickly realized that I was wrong—I was not as close to forgiving as I'd thought. I'm not a violent person, but my fist clenched as he drew near. The anger again shot through me. The nurse and Adam had already moved off the elevator, and the nurse spoke up,

"Ron, are you coming?" I walked off.

I am committed to forgiving, and I'm making progress. But it isn't like flipping a switch. It is one more ongoing struggle. I realize that Dr. Kay didn't go in to work that day intending to kill a patient. His job isn't easy. (That's why I design cabinets. Nobody dies from a bad cabinet.) But the emotions remain hard to control. I'm convinced, though, that I'll get there—with God's grace.

Just in case you're wondering how we're doing today. Our youngest son Clay is almost thirteen and a very active kid. He still enjoys playing basketball, and wants to play football next year. Clay is a lot closer with his mother as Adam is. Troy is now fourteen, and more of a dad's boy. He enjoys being in Scouts and being in track. I've taken responsibility for forming them in Catholicism, and that's been rewarding for us. Adam and Emily are about to get married in a few weeks. Adam is living in an apartment in town. He and Emily are both getting close to graduating college. Emily is working at a local hospital, and Adam is working part-time at a local furniture store. Isaiah is now 4 years old and is gearing up to go to school next year. He keeps himself pretty busy farming with his little tractors and farm equipment. They were all very frightened when we almost "lost" one another, and we've come closer together through the experience. I can't even imagine how I would have felt if my dad had nearly died when I was young. I hate to think how scared my family and loved ones were, because I know I was terrified.

Tina is still working her factory job. However, she got breast cancer in mid 2019. She did several treatments of radiation, and is currently in remission. She's still in some discomfort from her breast cancer, but is fine overall. Like most cancer survivors, she does her yearly check-ups. Unfortunately, she lost her mother a few months ago. So, she's trying to get through those emotions also.

As for me, I'm still working at my architecture job. I too go to get my cancer check-ups. Health problems are still a part of my life. About a year ago, I had yet another surgery to repair the damage in my stomach, so I could return to normal eating and digestive habits. It went well and I am continuing to improve each day. I had quite a bit of pain and irritation in my stomach after the first few surgeries three years ago. Today, I have a loss of feeling in my stomach and pain once in a while. The lead doctor who literally saved my life in 2017 also performed my surgery on December 3, 2019. He said that I can expect to have most of the feeling in my stomach return over time, possibly within the next year. The biggest downside to all of my health issues that I went through is probably the PTSD. It typically gets pretty difficult. But it's OK because I'm here. Like my oldest sister always told Caleb and me, "Somebody always has it worse than we do." The older I've gotten, and the more I see in life, the more I realize how true that really is.

Other than that, I continue to read my Bible every day and do my best to follow God's teachings.

Tina and I are still working on our relationship. It has improved since my health crisis—in part because I've abandoned the bad habits that were aggravating tensions—but married life continues to have its ups and downs. We have a tendency to escalate any differences into major conflicts, and we need to form new habits. Becoming more serious about my faith has been a blessing to me. After all, if there's a family that has a great deal to be thankful for, it's ours. We are committed to our union, and we continue to hope that we can reach a state that can truly be described as a "happy marriage."

A Final Plea

If you read nothing else in this book, I hope you will read these final comments.

Please don't make the same mistake that I made. Don't take life for granted. Not everyone gets a second chance like I did.

Life can be a struggle at times. No one should be surprised at that. Every year, I watch the movie *The Passion of the Christ.* I love that movie, and I hate it. When I watch it, I get angry and I have to walk away from the TV screen. What Jesus went through on our behalf is shocking. I know that my suffering is nothing compared to what His was. Our Father's grace was with Him to get Him through it all, and I know that He will be with me to get me through it all, too. I fall all the time. But I know that no matter how many times you fall, God is there to help you get back up. That's one of the lessons that sank deeply into me the day that changed my life. God sent His only Son to save me.

I never thought I would write a book, but God put it on my heart to do so, and He put me in touch with people who could help me make it happen. I believe that God wants this story to get out there so people know that he is real. He wants me to be an instrument for this message: that people can beat anything in accordance with God's will. It might be family conflict, cancer, botched surgeries, or anything else. We all experience challenges of some kind, or we accompany others when they do. God is by our side through it all.

In conclusion, though life was amazing growing up, I made mistakes. I left the Church. I made selfish decisions, but then, I gave myself to God. Who knows, maybe that's why the Lord saved me, why He gave me the "second chance" that I begged him for. Many people at the hospital told me that I shouldn't have survived what I did. I know it was only possible through God. There is no way I could have lived through it on my own.

I'm an example of how people can change. You can, just like I have. You don't need a near-death experience to do it. My outlook on life is different from what it was before my health crisis. I see things in a completely new light. It's like I took a big step back and God gave me a new pair of glasses. I'm not perfect. I just try to be a better person and to help others when I can. Christ tells us, "Love your neighbor as yourself" (Mark 12: 31). I've tried to take that command more seriously, and I encourage you to do the same.

God is real and He loves us. If a battle of some kind has made its way into your life, then He will give you the strength to fight. In fact, He won't just give you the strength; He will be your strength.

Make the most of your life and your circumstance. I needed a second chance to do that, but my hope and my prayer is that you won't. Don't delay. Start living your second chance now. May God bless each and every one of you.

Finally, I want to thank you for purchasing this book. May God bless you and keep you healthy.